THE KETOGENIC DIET FOR BEGINNERS

21 DAYS TO RAPID FAT LOSS

Mark G.Moore

TABLE OF CONTENTS

Warning

Remember that this is only a guide for informational purposes, we are not responsible for any physical or other damage. In case you wish to practice this type of nutrition, we advise you to contact a doctor.

INTRODUCTION

Are you a meat lover but need to lose weight? Then you might find yourself in a dilemma as most diets out there limit the intake of meat and other fatty food products because of high-fat content and calories as well. With that said, people who need to lose weight no longer have to be contented with eating carrot sticks or lettuce as one can now enjoy their favorite bacon and egg while still losing weight. The ketogenic diet, which once served as an epileptic prevention meal plan, is now being used by people who need to shed excess weight.

Some would argue that only the first "phase" of the Atkins Diet is "ketogenic" but it's very clear that this element is central to the whole diet. There are many other diets of this type with different names and claims but, if they talk about severely restricting the intake of carbohydrates, then they're probably forms of ketogenic diet. The process of "ketosis" is quite complicated and would take some time to describe but, in essence, it works because cutting down on carbs restricts the amount of blood glucose available to trigger the "insulin response". Without a triggering of the glucose-insulin response, some hormonal changes take place which causes the body to start burning its stores of fat as energy. This also has the interesting effect of causing your brain to be fuelled by what is known as "ketone bodies" (hence "ketogenic") rather than the usual glucose. The whole process is really quite fascinating and I recommend that you read up on it.

All forms of the ketogenic diet are controversial. Most of the debate surrounds the issue of cholesterol and whether ketogenic diets increase or decrease the levels HDL "good" cholesterol and/or increase or decrease LDL "bad" cholesterol. The number of scientific studies is increasing year on year and it is certainly possible to point to strong cases on both sides of the argument. My general conclusion is that one could equally make the case that a carbohydrate-laden diet has negative effects on cholesterol and I think that, on balance, a ketogenic-type diet is healthier than a carbohydrate-heavy one. Interestingly, there isn't so much controversy about whether ketogenic diets work or not (it's widely accepted that they do); it's mostly about how they work and whether that is good/bad/indifferent from a health perspective.

CHAPTER ONE
WHAT THE DIET IS?

The word "diet" has been a popular term since the 20th century when many weight loss techniques and advancements in health and nutrition were introduced. Through the years, several connotations of the term have evolved and a number of people are confused about the true meaning of the word. This is why it is very important for everyone to know what a diet is and to understand its nature.

Diet basically refers to all of the food that a person eats or consumes for a specific period of time.

A healthy and balanced diet requires a person to consume right amounts of food from each food group. The food pyramid is a good basis for knowing how much food from each food group a person has to consume each day. Following the food, pyramid balances our food consumption and eliminates the chances of overeating food from a particular food group. On the other hand, a poor diet mainly sticks to one specific food group. Poor diets eventually lead to vitamin and mineral deficiencies. It is not enough for a person to know the real meaning of the word "diet," but it is of equal importance to understand what a diet is for.

Diets may have several purposes and may come in different forms.

Contrary to popular belief, the regulation of diets is not only for weight loss, but it can also make people gain weight. Those who want to lose weight may opt to conform to a low-fat diet, in which fruits and vegetables are one of the dominant components. People who want to gain weight, on the other hand, may go for high-carbohydrate diets.

When a person is asked the question "What is a diet?" the first thing that usually comes to mind is weight loss.

There are more people who regulate their diets for the purpose of losing weight than those who want to increase their kilograms. This is the reason why diets tend to be more popularly thought of as a regimen that can help people reduce weight. A lot of weight loss diets have been introduced and have evolved in the field of nutrition and many of these are proven to be very effective. Unconventional weight loss diets have also emerged; an example is a liquid diet in which low-calorie beverages have to be consumed by weight losers on a regular basis.

For people who are naturally skinny or for those who are suffering from illnesses that cause drastic weight loss, a protein-rich diet is highly recommended. Protein is known to build muscles, thus resulting in weight gain. This is also the kind of diet that is suggested to bodybuilders for them to maintain their current figure and weight.

Diets are undoubtedly one of the trends nowadays, so everyone has to know what a diet is, what its functions are, and what its different forms are. This way, people would not just undergo a fad diet without proper consultation, causing health and body problems. Before starting a diet, a person must research about that particular diet or consult an expert first to ensure that it is safe and that he will be getting the most out of the regimen.

THE KETOGENIC DIET

The ketogenic diet is a low carb, moderate protein, and high-fat diet which put the body into a metabolic state known as ketosis. That's a pretty boring description but it is accurate. Essentially what this means is that when you figure out your macros (more on that later) then you'll find that you're eating mostly fats (these are good for you), some protein, and very little crabs.

Getting into ketosis is the goal of the ketogenic diet.

When you're the body is in a state of ketosis, the liver produces ketones which become the main energy source for the body and this all revolves around the consumption of fat. This can be a complete mind twist for some people because "fat" just isn't a good word but your body loves to live off of healthy fats. We'll talk more about this later on. The ketogenic diet is also referred to as keto (key-toe) diet, low carb diet, and low carb high fat (LCHF).

So why is it so awesome and why is it taking the world by storm?

Because it completely reverses how your body functions (in a good way) along with changing how you view nutrition. If you have decided to lose weight this spring, then you might want to consider the Ketogenic diet.

The diet has been around for a long time and was once used to treat patients with epileptic or seizure problems, especially among young kids. Nowadays, the diet has lost its popularity with the advent of prescription drugs that treat the health problem.

The diet, however, is used by many dieters around the world because of its efficacy and although diets have its side effects, knowing about the diet and following the rules can help one lose weight without compromising their overall health. As always, those with health problems should consult their medical health provider so that they can help patients to adjust to the meal plan or to monitor them to ensure that the ketogenic therapy will not affect their health.

SEVEN TIPS FOR GETTING INTO KETOSIS.

1. Minimize your carb intake to 25-50 net carbs a day

2. Include coconut oil in your diet

3. Ramp up your physical activity

4. Increase healthy fats

5. Short periods of fasting

6. Maintain protein intake

7. Test ketones levels

If you are considering these dietary changes, it is always recommended that you check with your physician. Keto is a lifestyle change. You are changing the way you eat. In order for you to gain success, you should be consistent and consider the long-term consequences.

RULES OF THE DIET

1. Never skip breakfast

The old saying that 'breakfast is the most important meal of the day' is certainly on the money when it comes to dieting. Nothing gets our metabolism going faster than breakfast after a good night's sleep.

Sleeping causes our metabolism to slow right down and breakfast kick-starts it again for us. But always remember that just as important as having breakfast itself, it's also important to choose healthy breakfast options like wholegrain cereals and bread, low-fat dairy products like milk and yogurt, and fruit or fruit juice.

2. Drink plenty of water

Drinking plenty of water is critically important when we are dieting. As well as helping to keep us healthy, drinking sufficient amounts of water can help us when dieting because it helps keep us feeling full and stops us from feeling hungry, and when we drink plenty of water we usually drink less soda, coffee, and alcohol, all of which can add significant amounts of calories to our daily intake.3.

3. Count your calories

Do you know how many calories you need to maintain your current weight and do you know how many calories you, therefore, need to consume in order to lose weight?

Once you know these things, you also need to keep track of how many calories you consume each day so that you can compare them to your target and make any necessary adjustments.

Writing down your calorie consumption after each meal will help you realize how much of an effect the little piece of chocolate here and the occasional cookie there has on your weight.

4. Don't try to lose weight quickly

Gaining significant weight usually takes years and so should lose a significant amount of weight. Our bodies don't like sudden and significant change; in fact, it is built to resist it.

This resistance has a scientific name called homeostasis. When our body heats up to a temperature above its preferred level what happens? We sweat, which an automatic response is designed to cool us down to the preferred level again. That's homeostasis at work. When we lose weight too quickly, what happens? Our body automatically slows down its metabolism, that is, the rate at which we burn energy to survive and function. That's homeostasis at work again.

In addition to keeping our body from fighting against us on the weight loss front, losing weight too quickly doesn't work because early rapid weight loss usually results from losing body fluid and muscle tissue which is not healthy nor helpful in our battle to lose weight.

5. It's not just what you eat that counts

Weight gain isn't a sign that we have been eating the wrong food; it is a sign that we have been eating too much food. The great news about this is that we don't need to all start eating lettuce to lose weight; we just may need to cut down a little on the foods we enjoy each day.

6. Keeping your metabolism up

Muscle and activity keep our metabolism up which is why weight training to build or maintain our muscle mass and aerobic activity like walking, jogging, cycling, and swimming are so important to those of us wanting to lose weight.

Dieting alone is not the best route to weight loss and to staying in an ideal weight range. To lose weight safely and keep it off for as long as possible, always combine dieting and exercise.

7. You won't continue to eat foods you don't like

Most diets fail because they require us to eat plenty of foods we don't actually like. If we don't like what we're eating we're not going to stick with our diet for more than a week or two. The key to successful dieting is to reduce the amount we eat and introduce healthier and lower calorie options of the foods we like gradually into our diet over time.

8. Watch what you drink as well as eat

Almost everything we drink, except water, has calories in it.

Drinks highest in calories are typically sodas, colas, and alcoholic drinks.

If we usually drink a lot of any of these high-calorie drinks, it may be them and not what we're eating that is causing us to get fat.

9. Avoid extremes of any kind

Balance is not only the key to a happy, healthy life; it is also the key to a healthy diet and dieting.

Be wary of any diets that completely cut out some

foods or food groups or that severely limit some foods or food groups, for example very low or no-carb diets. Diets that are extreme in one way or another are likely to be very unhealthy at best and very dangerous to our health at worst.

10. Get help

If you have a lot of weight to lose, you've got a better chance of success if you get help. If your weight is affecting your health to such an extent that it is or is becoming life-threatening or is leading to you suffering from weight-related diseases like type-2 diabetes, seek medical help from a doctor or professional help from a dietician or another suitably qualified health care professional to lose weight immediately.

Some would argue that only the first "phase" of the Atkins Diet is "ketogenic" but it's very clear that this element is central to the whole diet. There are many other diets of this type with different names and claims but, if they talk about severely restricting the intake of carbohydrates, then they're probably forms of ketogenic diet. The process of "ketosis" is quite complicated and would take some time to describe but, in essence, it works because cutting down on carbs restricts the amount of blood glucose available to trigger the "insulin response".

Without a triggering of the glucose-insulin response, some hormonal changes take place which causes the body to start burning its stores of fat as energy. This also has the interesting effect of causing your brain to be fuelled by what is known as "ketone bodies" (hence "ketogenic") rather than the usual glucose. The whole process is really quite fascinating and I recommend that you read up on it.

CHAPTER TWO
FACTS BEHIND THE KETOGENIC DIET

There are many diets in the world, and often people will engage in radical behavior or follow extreme diets without becoming aware of the biological and physiological consequences of their actions. Fasting was one such diet that was at first practiced for theoretical beliefs in purity, abstinence and such, and only after were the biological processes at play understood, researched, the practice refined. What was discovered is that fasting produces the same results as a carbohydrate free diet and that by restricting the carbs in your diet you can achieve rapid weight loss.

This approach is called the ketogenic diet, and it is so named because the form of abstinence from carbs causes bodies called ketones to be produced by the liver, which then helps your body process fat as a primary source of energy instead of glucose. Why is that?

Traditionally our bodies burn glucose as our primary form of fuel. Glucose is derived from carbohydrates, with excess glucose getting stored in the muscles and liver as glycogen. What excess glucose remains after that process is then turned into fat. When we cut all carbs from our diet, we no longer have access to glucose, which forces our bodies to burn through the glycogen reserves and then start oxidizing fat. This would be fine but for the fact that certain tissues such as parts of our brain can only be sustained by glucose, which is where ketone production comes in.

The production of ketones allows those tissues to substitute ketones for glucose and allow us to survive without any carbs at all. If you eat less than 100 grams per day you will trigger this process, resulting in a diet that is based solely on fat and protein and which burns fat and protein as a source of fuel. Unless managed correctly, such a diet can cause your body to cannibalize your lean body mass as well as your fat, resulting in a dramatic drop in weight that cannot be wholly attributed to fat loss.

Where do ketones come from? They are produced by the liver as a by-product of free fatty acid breakdown. Ketones are thus derived from fat, and their production also has consequences on the hormone levels in your body which are normally used to regulate glucose movement in your bloodstream such as insulin.

That is why many people report feeling sluggish or exhausted when on the ketogenic diet.

DO KETOGENIC DIETS WORK

It's long been established in scientific circles that blood sugar was taken from food is absolutely vital for survival. Without it, a person will become sick, weak, and eventually die. However, in the past few decades, many bodybuilders have chosen to be 'guinea pigs' for their own analysis into what happens when carbohydrates - the means for bringing blood sugar into the body - are removed. The results were twofold. First, the bodybuilders achieved new levels of muscularity and conditioning. Second, they did not die, despite the scientific belief that it was impossible to maintain blood sugar levels without eating carbohydrates.

It turns out that the liver creates new blood sugar. It takes components of lactic acid and pyruvic acid which exist in the body and combines them with amino acids which enter the body through consumption of protein foods (or amino acid supplements). The liver forms new glycogen (blood sugar) at higher levels than it is consuming. Remember, the liver regularly breaks down glycogen as part of its normal routine.

In terms of effectiveness, ketogenic (low-carb) diets can be very beneficial for bodybuilders of the intermediate or advanced level, who already possess a decent amount of muscle mass. It is very hard to gain muscle while not consuming carbohydrates. Ketogenic diets are very effective because they force your body to consume fat stores for energy, instead of choosing to utilize the sugars in your blood from your daily carb consumption. There are side effects, and they are compounded greatly to negative effect when the bodybuilder doesn't consume adequate fiber through supplementation or daily no-carb vegetable ingestion.

The bottom line is that ketogenic diets are very effective for burning body fat, as long as they are done correctly. Ketogenic dieting defies scientific rationale, and there is still a great deal unknown about the long-term effects of low-carbohydrate dieting. Research it, and you might find that it's right for you when the next pre-contest diet begins.

MAKING KETOGENIC DIETS WORK

Ketogenic Diets are the most effective diets for achieving rapid, ultra low body fat levels with maximum muscle retention! Now, as with all such general statements, there are circumstantial exceptions. But done right - which they rarely are - the fat loss achievable on a ketogenic diet is nothing short of staggering! And, despite what people might tell you, you will also enjoy the incredibly high energy and overall sense of well being.

THE PERCEPTION

Despite these promises, more bodybuilders/shapers have had negative experiences that have seen positive results. The main criticisms are:

- Chronic lethargy

- Unbearable hunger

- Massive decrease in gym performance

- Severe muscle loss

All of these criticisms result from a failure to heed the caveat above: Ketogenic Diets must be done right! It must be realized that they are an entirely unique metabolic modality that adheres to none of the previously accepted 'rules' of dieting. And there is no going halfway; 50 grams of carbs per day plus high protein intake is not ketogenic.

So how ketogenic are diets 'done right'? Let's quickly look at how they work.

Simply, our body, organs, muscles, and brain can use either glucose or ketones for fuel. It is the function of the liver and pancreas (primarily) to regulate that fuel supply and they show a strong bias toward sticking with glucose. Glucose is the 'preferred' fuel because it is derived in abundance from the diet and readily available readily from liver and muscle stores.

Ketones have to be deliberately synthesized by the liver, but the liver can easily synthesize glucose (a process known as 'gluconeogenesis' that uses amino acids (protein) or other metabolic intermediaries) too.

We don't get beta hydroxybutyrate, acetone, or acetoacetate (ketones) from the diet. The liver synthesizes them only under duress; as a last measure in conditions of severe glucose deprivation like starvation. For the liver to be convinced that ketones are the order of the day, several conditions must be met:

- Blood glucose must fall below 50mg/dl

- Low blood glucose must result in low Insulin and elevated Glucagon

- Liver glycogen must be low or 'empty'

- A plentiful supply of gluconeogenic substrates must not be available

At this point it is important to mention that it is not actually a question of being 'in' or 'out' of ketosis; we don't either totally run on ketones, or not. It is a gradual and careful transition so that the brain is constantly and evenly fuelled... ideally. Ketones should be produced in small amounts from blood glucose levels of about 60mg/dl. We consider ourselves in ketosis when there are greater concentrations of ketones than glucose in the blood.

The reality is that most people - especially weight trainers - have had a regular intake of glucose for a good couple of decades, at least. The liver is perfectly capable of producing ketones but the highly efficient gluconeogenic pathways are able to maintain low-normal blood glucose above the ketogenic threshold.

Couple this with the fact that many people are at least partially insulin resistant and have elevated fasting insulin (upper end of the normal range, anyway). The small amount of blood glucose from gluconeogenesis induces sufficient insulin release to blunt glucagon output and the production of ketones.

Sudden glucose deprivation will have the consequence, initially, of lethargy, hunger, weakness etc in most people - until ketosis is achieved. And Ketosis will not be reached until the liver is forced to quit with gluconeogenesis and start producing ketones. As long as dietary protein is sufficient then the liver will continue to produce glucose and not ketones. That's why no carb, high protein diets are not ketogenic.

WHAT'S SO GREAT ABOUT KETOSIS?

When the body switches over to running primarily on ketones a number of very cool things happen:

•	Lipolysis (body fat breakdown) is substantially increased

•	Muscle catabolism (muscle loss) is substantially reduced

•	Energy levels are maintained in a high and stable state

- Subcutaneous fluid (aka 'water retention') is eliminated

Basically, when we are in ketosis our body is using fat (ketones) to fuel everything. As such, we aren't breaking down muscle to provide glucose. That is, muscle is being spared because it has nothing to offer; fat is all the body needs (well, to a large extent). For the dieter, this means substantially less muscle loss than what is achievable on any other diet. Make sense?

As a bonus, ketones yield only 7 calories per gram. This is higher than the equal mass of glucose but substantially less (22%, in fact) than the 9 calorie gram of fat from whence it came. We like metabolic inefficiencies like this. They mean we can eat more but the body doesn't get the calories.

Even cooler is that ketones cannot be turned back into fatty acids; the body excretes any excess in the urine! Speaking of which, there will be quite a bit of urine; the drop in muscle glycogen, low Insulin, and low aldosterone all equate to massive excretion of intra and extracellular fluid. For us that means hard, defined muscularity and quick, visible results.

Regarding energy, our brain actually really likes ketones so we tend to feel fantastic in ketosis - clear headed, alert and positive. And because there is never a shortage of fat to supply ketones, energy is high all the time. Usually, you even sleep less and wake feeling more refreshed when in ketosis.

DOING IT RIGHT

From what's said above you will realize that to get into ketosis:

- Carbohydrate intake should be ZERO

- Protein intake should be low - 25% of calories at a maximum

- Fat must account for 75%+ of calories

With low insulin (due to zero carbs) and calories at, or below maintenance, the dietary fat cannot be deposited in adipose tissues. The low protein means that gluconeogenesis will quickly prove inadequate to maintain blood glucose and, whether the body likes it or not, there is still all the damned fat to burn.

And burn it does. The high dietary fat is oxidized for cellular energy in the normal fashion but winds up generating quantities of Acetyl-CoA that exceed the capacity of the TCA cycle. The significant result is ketogenesis - a synthesis of ketones from the excess Acetyl-CoA. In more lay terms: the high fat intake "forces" ketosis upon the body. This is how it's 'done right'.

Now you just have to throw out what you thought was true about fats. Firstly, fat does not 'make you fat". Most of the information about the evils of saturated fats, in particular, is so disproportionate or plain wrong anyway; on a ketogenic diet, it is doubly inapplicable. Saturated fats make ketosis fly.

And don't worry; your heart will be better than fine and your insulin sensitivity will not be reduced (there is no insulin around in the first place)!

Once in ketosis, it is not necessary, technically speaking, to maintain absolute zero carbs or low protein. But it is still better if you want to reap the greatest rewards. Besides, assuming you are training hard, you will still want to follow a cyclic ketogenic diet where you get to eat all your carbs, fruit and whatever else, every 1-2 weeks.

Don't be mistaken; 'done right' does not make ketogenic dieting easy or fun for the culinary acrobats among you. They are probably the most restrictive diets you can use and not an option if you don't love animal products. Get out your nutritional almanac and work out a 20:0:80 protein: carb: fat diet. Yeah, it's boring. As an example, your daily ketogenic diet is 3100 Calories at 25:0.5:74.5 from only:

- 10 xxl Whole Eggs

- 160ml Pure Cream (40% fat)

- 400g Mince (15% fats)

- 60ml Flaxseed Oil

- 30g Whey Protein Isolate

Ketogenic diets offer a host of unique benefits that cannot be ignored if you are chasing the ultimate, low body fat figure or physique. However, they are not the most user's friendly of diets and any 'middle ground' compromise you might prefer will be just the worst of all worlds. Your choice is to do them right or not at all.

CHAPTER THREE
KETOGENIC DIET PLAN EXPLAINED

For the best diet to rapidly burn fat using the body's natural metabolism, consider a ketogenic diet plan. Nutrition has the strongest effect on the body's production of important hormones, which regulate metabolism and allow the body to burn fat for energy and retain muscle mass, with little need for excessive exercise.

WHAT IS A KETOGENIC DIET PLAN?

Basically, it is a diet that causes the body to enter a state of ketosis. Ketosis is a natural and healthy metabolic state in which the body burns its own stored fat (producing ketones), instead of using glucose (the sugars from carbohydrates found in the Standard American Diet - SAD). Metabolically speaking, ketogenic foods are very powerful. The amazing benefit is that these foods are also delicious, natural whole foods that are extremely healthy for you.

Some of the best-tasting, most fulfilling foods are part of this plan, including lean meats like beef and chicken, healthy sources of protein and high-quality fats like eggs, butter, olive oil, coconut oil, and avocado. Also, delicious leafy-green vegetables like kale, chard, and spinach, as well as cruciferous vegetables like broccoli, cabbage, and cauliflower.

These foods can be combined with seeds, nuts, sprouts, and a wide range of other amazing foods that lead to incredible health benefits that give your body the protein, healthy fats, and nutrients it needs while providing metabolism-boosting meals for easy cooking at home or on the go.

KETOGENIC DIET PLAN WHAT FOODS SHOULD BE LIMITED?

On a ketogenic diet plan, the main foods to avoid are those high in carbohydrates, sugars, and the wrong types of fats. These foods can be toxic to the body and create excess glucose levels that the body turns into stored fat.

These foods increase the level of insulin and blood sugar in the body and will prevent fat loss even if you are putting a lot of energy into exercise. To avoid these foods, limit your intake of grains, processed foods, vegetable oils (canola, corn, soybean, etc.), milk, margarine, and other high-carbohydrate, high-sugar foods.

We have been told for decades that calories from fats should be reduced to encourage weight loss, but this is a vast over-simplification (still supported by government and industrial food interests) that is no longer accurate according to our modern understanding of human nutrition. The reality is that certain fats are not good for you (those high in omega-6 fatty acids) because your body has a hard time processing them. Other fats, particularly medium chain triglycerides (MCTs), are extremely beneficial for weight loss, brain cell generation, and nutrients. These healthy saturated fats should be increased to give your body the energy it needs while in ketosis while limiting the detrimental trans-fats found in many processed foods.

KETOGENIC DIET PLAN

Recent studies have demonstrated that a higher protein, low carbohydrate diet promotes superior results for fat loss, improvements in blood lipid parameters and increased thermogenesis in individuals with obesity and insulin resistance and may help to resolve the metabolic blocks that can prevent fat loss. The Ketogenic diet involves significantly reducing carbohydrate intake while increasing protein to the levels necessary to maintain muscle mass with the calorie ratios approximating 50% protein, 20% low glycemic index carbohydrates and 30% therapeutic fats.

The general dietary guidelines involve avoidance of high carbohydrate foods such as bread, pasta, potatoes, rice etc. as well as all simple carbohydrates such as sugar, honey, and fruit juice.

Protein is included in every meal as this helps to reduce appetite, regulate blood glucose levels and preserve lean muscle mass.

Examples of protein foods are fish, chicken, turkey, meat, eggs, cheese, tofu, and tempeh. Protein drinks such as whey protein isolate or soy protein may be utilized. Soy protein is especially beneficial as it has been shown to stimulate thyroid hormone production, reduce fat levels and promote fat loss, due to the phytoestrogens and essential fatty acids it contains.

Adequate fat intake is also essential as this enhances fat burning by the body while reducing the synthesis of fatty acids in the body which both promote fat loss.

Optimal sources of fats are flaxseed oil, fish oil, avocado, olive oil, nuts, and seeds.

To provide balanced nutrition, vitamins, minerals, and fiber and to promote detoxification it is also essential to consume 3-4 cups of low carbohydrate vegetables or salad daily with one optional serve of fresh fruit daily.

When beginning a Ketogenic diet program some discomfort may be experienced such as headaches, irritability, fatigue, and hunger for the first 2-7 days, however thereafter it is very easy to adhere to the diet and it actually reduces appetite, carbohydrate cravings and increases energy levels.

A TYPICAL DAY ON THE KETOGENIC DIET MAY BE AS FOLLOWS:

BREAKFAST

- Scrambled eggs or tofu with parsley, scallions, spinach, and tomato OR

- Protein powder blended with fresh or frozen berries

LUNCH

- Salad with tuna/salmon/eggs/cottage cheese

DINNER

- Fish, chicken, turkey, tofu or meat with steamed or stir fried low carbohydrate vegetables

- Snacks: (2-3 daily)

- Protein drink OR

- Hardboiled egg OR

- Handful of nuts or seeds

The Ketogenic diet produces very good results when followed consistently. Long term success is more likely if a holistic attitude is adopted that addresses diet, exercise, nutritional supplements, and psychological factors as well as any specific health challenges that are unique to the individual.

When the ideal body fat percentage is achieved the diet may be gradually adjusted to include more complex carbohydrates such as whole grains, starchy vegetables, and fruit while as much as possible avoiding all other simple carbohydrates such as sugar, honey, and refined flours. Simultaneously it is essential to ensure that protein is included in every meal.

This more relaxed type of dietary approach can be maintained indefinitely in conjunction with a regular exercise program to ensure that body weight and composition remains stable.

WHY KETOGENIC DIET?

1.   Burn Stored Fat: By cutting out the high levels of carbohydrates in your diet that produce glucose (sugar), a ketogenic diet plan tells your body to burn stored fat by converting this fat into fatty acids and ketone bodies in the liver. These ketone bodies replace the role of glucose that was being filled by carbohydrates in the diet. This leads to a rapid reduction in the amount of fat stored in the body.

2.   Retain Muscle Mass: By including the right fats in your diet, a ketogenic diet plan provides your body with the energy it needs to convert

existing fat stores into useful sugars and ketones (through gluconeogenesis), which are an essential source of energy for the brain, muscles, and heart. This has the added benefit of preserving muscle mass because the healthy fat in the diet gives the body the energy it needs without having to tap into muscle protein to create more sugar. This creates the best of both worlds - burn fat while maintaining muscle mass!

3.   Eliminate Excess Fat: Even better, if your body creates too many ketone bodies by converting existing fat, it will simply eliminate

those ketones as a waste product, which means you will basically pee out unwanted body fat.

4.   Reduce Appetite: By regulating the powerful metabolic hormones in your body, a ketogenic diet plan will actually reduce your appetite. By lowering your body's insulin resistance and increasing ketones, you will actually feel less hungry on this diet, which is an amazing advantage over other low-calorie, carbohydrate-rich weight loss diets that come with the expectation of lingering hunger.

Start burning fat today without more exercise! Take control of your metabolism naturally by adopting a ketogenic diet plan. Your body was designed for this style of nutrition. Your metabolic state can be optimized by consuming the (delicious) foods that our genetic forefathers thrived on, and this does not include carbohydrate-rich, processed foods loaded with sugars and bad fats. It involves a luxurious and fulfilling diet based on bountiful foods from Paleolithic times, including lean meats, vegetables, nuts and seeds, and healthy fats that your body will thank you for.

CHAPTER FOUR
HISTORY OF THE RAPID WEIGHT LOSS EFFECTS OF KETOGENIC DIETS

Virtually all weight loss diets to varying degrees focus on either calorie reduction or the manipulation of the intake of one of the three essential macronutrients (proteins, fats, or carbohydrates) to achieve their weight loss effects.

Ketogenic diets are a group of "high-fat, moderate protein" or "high-protein moderate fat" but very low-carbohydrate diets.

The first sets of ketogenic diets were actually developed as far back as the early 1920s by the

Johns Hopkins Pediatric Epilepsy Center and also by Dr. R.M. Wilder of the Mayo Clinic to treat children with hard to control seizures. The diets were designed to mimic the biochemical changes that occurred during periods of fasting, namely ketosis, acidosis, and dehydration. The diets involved the consumption of about 10-15 grams of carbohydrates per day, 1 gram of protein per kilogram body weight of the patient and the remaining calories derived from fats.

Today, the promoters of ketogenic diets are strong of the view that carbohydrates especially the high glycemic index ones are the major reasons why people gain weight. Carbohydrate foods are generally metabolized to produce glucose, a form of simple sugar that is generally regarded as the preferred energy source for the body as it is a faster burning energy.

Although the body can break down muscle glycogen (a mixture of glucose and water) and fat to produce energy, it, however, prefers to get it from high glycemic index carbohydrates from diets.

Of the macronutrients, carbohydrates are therefore argued to be the major cause of weight gain. This is more so because the increased intake of high glycemic index carbohydrate foods generally causes fluctuating blood sugar levels due to their fast absorption into the bloodstream and which more often than not leads to the overproduction of insulin. This is where the problem actually starts.

Insulin is a hormone that regulates blood glucose levels and therefore maintenance of the energy in/energy out the equation of the body which rules body weight.

Excess amounts of glucose in the bloodstream causes the excessive secretion of insulin which leads to the storage of the excess glucose in the body as either glycogen in liver and muscle cells or fat in fat cells.

One aim of ketogenic diets is, therefore, to reduce insulin production to its barest minimum by drastically reducing carbohydrate consumption while using fats and proteins to supplement the body's energy requirement.

Despite the ability of ketogenic diets to reduce insulin production, their main objective is ultimately aimed at inducing the state of ketosis. Ketosis can be regarded as a condition or state in which the rate of formation of ketones produced by the breakdown of "fat" into "fatty acids" by the liver is greater than the ability of tissues to oxidize them. Ketosis is actually a secondary state of the process of lipolysis (fat break down) and is a general side effect of low-carbohydrate diets. Ketogenic diets are therefore favorably disposed to the encouragement and promotion of ketosis.

Prolonged periods of starvation can easily induce ketosis but it can also be deliberately induced by making use of a low-calorie or low-carbohydrate diet through the ingestion of large amounts of either fats or proteins and drastically reduced carbohydrates.

Therefore, high-fat and high-protein diets are the weight loss diets used to deliberately induce ketosis.

Essentially, ketosis is a very efficient form of energy production which does not involve the production of insulin as the body rather burns its fat deposits for energy. Consequently, the idea of reducing carbohydrate consumption does not only reduce insulin production but also practically forces the body to burn its fat deposit for energy, thereby making the use of ketogenic diets a very powerful way to achieve rapid weight loss.

Ketogenic diets are designed in such a way that they initially force the body to exhaust its glucose supply and then finally switch to burning its fat deposits for energy.

Subsequent food intakes after inducing the state of ketosis are meant to keep the ketosis process running by appropriately adjusting further carbohydrate consumption to provide just the basic amount of calories needed by the body.

For example, the Atkins Diet which is obviously the most popular ketogenic diet aims to help dieters achieve what the diet calls the individual's Critical Carbohydrate Level for Maintenance

(CCLM) - a carbohydrate consumption level where the dieter neither gains nor loses weight anymore.

In 2003, the Johns Hopkins treatment center came up with a modified version of the Atkins Diet protocol to treat a group of 20 children with epilepsy. After the treatment, it was observed that two-thirds experienced a significant reduction in their seizures while 9 were able to reduce their medication dosages and none developed kidney stones.

CHAPTER FIVE
KETOGENIC DIET MENU FOR THE BEGINNER

If you have decided to lose weight, then you might want to consider the Ketogenic diet. The diet has been around for a long time and was once used to treat patients with epileptic or seizure problems, especially among young kids as started in chapter two. Nowadays, the diet has lost its popularity with the advent of prescription drugs that treat the health problem. The diet, however, is used by many dieters around the world because of its efficacy, knowing about the diet and following the rules can help one lose weight without compromising their overall health.

Beginners especially should have a brief overview of the diet and the meal plan to help them make an informed decision should they decide to do the diet on their own. As always, those with health problems should consult their medical health provider so that they can help patients to adjust to the meal plan or to monitor them to ensure that the ketogenic therapy will not affect their health.

3 TYPES OF KETOGENIC DIETS

Ketogenic diet is a high fat low carbohydrate diet with adequate protein thrown in the meal. It is further divided into three types and depending on one's daily calorie needs, the percentage differs. Diets are often prepared on a ratio level such as 4:1 or 2:1 with the first number indicating the total fat amount in the diet compared to the protein and carbohydrate combined in each meal.

1.   STANDARD - SKD

The first diet is the Standard or the SKD and is designed for individuals who are not active or lead a sedentary lifestyle. The meal plan limits the dieter to eat a net of 20-50 grams of carbohydrates. Fruits or vegetables that are starchy are restricted from the diet. In order for the diet to be effective, one must strictly follow the meal plan. Butter, vegetable oil and heavy creams are used heavily to replace carbohydrates in the diet.

2.   TARGETED - TKD

The TKD is less strict than the SKD and allows one to consume carbohydrates though only in a certain portion or amount which will not impact the ketosis that one is currently in. The TKD diet helps dieters that perform some level of exercise or workout.

3.   CYCLICAL - CKD

The CKD is preferable for those who are into weight training or do intensive exercises and not for beginners as it requires the person undergoing the diet to stick to an SKD meal plan for the five days in a week's time and eating/loading up on carbohydrates on the next two days. It is important that dieters follow the strict regimen to ensure that their diet is successful.

The basis of many diets in the past was, "If you want to lose fat, you have to lower the fat intake to a minimum." That was also what the leading health institutes recommended. But in the last few years, that thesis was proven wrong. There are many scientific studies that show that we lose fat faster if we limit our carbohydrate consumption to a minimum, while increasing the fat intake.

The body needs energy for its activity. In general, the body gets this energy primary from carbohydrates, then fat and if necessary also from protein.

So if you limit the carbohydrate intake to 30grams or less, your body will have to search for an alternative fuel source, which is fat. Your body can still manufacture carbohydrates from protein and one of the components of fat (glycerol).

BODY ADJUSTMENT TO THE KETOGENIC DIET

The body needs three weeks to completely adjust to the usage of fatty acids and ketones as an energy source. If you try the ketogenic diet the first few days will be like hell, you will not be able to concentrate, you will be nauseous and weak.

This is because the body needs some time to adjust to the new energy source.

The body is used to carbohydrates and if you just lower your carbohydrate to zero, that will be a big shock. But when the body adjusts you will start benefiting from the ketogenic diet.

When you start eating high fat and low carbohydrate diet you will start influencing mainly two important hormones, insulin and glucagon. Insulin in the body transports nutrients from the blood to cells (like glucose to muscles). Glucagon acts as an opposite; it influences the cells to starts releasing the stored nutrients to the blood stream.

When there is a shortage of glucose it encourages the liver to produce glucose from other sources and releasing them into the blood, where they can reach any cell in the body.

If you lower the carbohydrate intake, the body gradually starts releasing less and less insulin and more glucagons. That and the small storage of carbohydrates in the blood soon start to release fatty acids from the fat deposits and transporting them to the liver where they are metabolized. That leads to increasing in ketone production, thereby putting the body in the state called ketosis.

CHAPTER SIX
TIPS FOR SUCCESS ON THE KETOGENIC DIET

Below are a few tips to maximize your success on a ketogenic diet.

1.   Drink tons of water.

While on a ketogenic diet, your body has a hard time retaining as much water as it needs, so staying properly hydrated is absolutely essential. Many experts recommend that men intake a minimum of 3 liters of beverages each day, while the figure for women is 2.2 liters daily. A good indicator of proper hydration is the color of your urine.

If your urine is clear or light yellow, you're most likely properly hydrated. Keep a bottle of water with you everywhere you go.

2.   Don't forget the fat

Simply put, our bodies need fuel to function. When we limit our carbohydrate intake, especially to levels that induce ketosis, our bodies need an alternate fuel source. Since protein is not an efficient source of energy, our bodies turn to fat. Any fat you eat while in ketosis is used for energy, making it very difficult to store fat while in ketosis.

Choose healthy, unsaturated fats as often as possible: foods like avocados, olives, nuts, and seeds are ideal.

3.   Find your carb limit.

All of our bodies are different. Some dieters will need to adhere to a strict low-carbohydrate diet that entails consuming less than 20 grams per day of carbs. Other dieters will find that they can comfortably stay in ketosis while consuming 50, 75, or 100 grams of carbohydrates. The only way to know for sure is trial and error. Purchase Ketosis or any brand of ketone urinalysis strips and find out your carbohydrate limit.

If you find that you have a bit of wiggle room, it will make sticking to your diet that much easier.

4.   Be smart about liquor.

One of the great aspects of the ketogenic diet is that you can drink liquor while on it without throwing your weight loss too far off course. You can drink unsweetened liquors like vodka, rum, tequila, gin, whiskey, scotch, cognac, and brandy, along with the occasional low-carb beer. Use low-carb mixers and drink plenty of water to stay hydrated, as hangovers are notoriously bad while in ketosis. And remember, calories still count, so don't go overboard. All things in moderation.

5.   Be patient.

While the ketogenic diet is known for rapid weight loss, especially in the early stages of the diet, weight loss is always a slow, time-consuming process. Don't freak out if the scale doesn't show weight loss, or shows slight weight increases, for a few days. Your weight varies day-to-day (and throughout the day) based upon a number of factors. Don't forget to use metrics like how your clothes fit or body measurements to see progress beyond what the scale shows.

CHAPTER SEVEN
KETOGENIC DIET BENEFITS OVER OTHER DIETS

1.   Being in ketosis allows the body to process fat and uses it as fuel in a way that no other state allows as easily. Carbohydrates are much easier to convert and use as fuel, so when you are providing plenty of these to your body, you need to burn and use all of those before your body will finally begin converting and using fat as fuel.

2.   Another benefit of being in a state of ketosis is that excess ketone is not harmful to your system in any way whatsoever. Any key tones that you create which are not needed by your body are

simply excreted through urine, easily and harmlessly. In fact, this excellent benefit is the reason why you can check whether you are in a state of ketosis using urine testing strips in the morning.

3.   When your body gets used to being in ketosis, it will actually begin to prefer ketones to glucose. This is the ideal state that you want your body to be in - no longer craving sugar whatsoever, and in fact preferring protein as a fuel source as opposed to sugar.

4.   Another benefit of ketogenic diet weight loss is that being in a ketogenic state is very useful

for controlling insulin levels in the body. Insulin is one of the substances that make you crave food, particularly for its high in sugar, and so controlling it to healthy levels is one of the key elements of weight loss.

5.   The majority of people who take advantage of ketogenic diet weight loss report that being in a ketogenic state makes them feel significantly less hungry than when they are in a non-ketogenic state. It is much easier to stick to a diet - any diet - when you're not fighting cravings and hunger every step of the way. In fact, hunger pangs can often be the thing that derails a person's best

efforts! Not having to deal with them makes it easier to meet your goals, all the way around.

Now that you are aware of all of the weight loss benefits of being in a state of ketosis, it makes sense that you would at least give this approach a try - after all, what do you have to lose except weight?

WHAT CAN I EAT ON A KETOGENIC DIET?

Here are some examples of high-fat low-carb foods on the ketogenic diet food list you can expect to eat lots of if you're following the ketogenic diet: Your keto meals should contain high amounts of healthy fats (up to 80 percent of your total calories!), such as olive oil, coconut oil, grass-fed butter, palm oil, and some nuts and seeds. Fats are a critical part of every ketogenic recipe because fat is what provides energy and prevents hunger, weakness, and fatigue. Keto meals also need all sorts of non-starchy vegetables. What vegetables can you eat on a ketogenic diet without worrying about increasing your carb intake too much? Some of the most popular choices include broccoli and other cruciferous veggies, all types of leafy greens, asparagus, cucumber, and zucchini.

In more moderate amounts, foods that are high in protein but low- or no-carb, including grass-fed meat, pasture-raised poultry, cage-free eggs, bone broth, wild-caught fish, organ meats and some full-fat (ideally raw) dairy products. On the other hand, the types of foods you'll avoid eating on the keto, low-carb diet are likely the same ones you are, or previously were, accustomed to getting lots of your daily calories from before starting this way of eating.

This includes items like fruit, processed foods or drinks high in sugar, those made with any grains or white/wheat flour, conventional dairy products, desserts, and many other high-carb foods (especially those that are sources of "empty calories").

Remember, that the goal of the ketogenic diet is to get your body into a state of ketosis and to do that you need to reduce your carb intake. It's important to understand that carbohydrates are not only in the junk foods that you love but also some of the healthier foods that you enjoy. For example, on keto, you need to avoid wheat (bread, pasta, cereals), starch (potatoes, beans, legumes) and fruit. There are small exceptions like avocado, star fruit, and berries as long as they are consumed in moderation.

SOME EXAMPLE OF FOODS TO AVOID

• Grains - wheat, corn, rice, cereal

• Sugar - honey, agave, maple syrup

• Fruit - apples, bananas, oranges

• Tubers - potato, yams

• Legumes

SOME EXAMPLE OF FOODS TO EAT

• Meats - fish, beef, lamb, poultry, egg

• Leafy Greens - spinach, kale

• Above ground vegetables - broccoli, cauliflower

• High-fat dairy - hard cheeses, high fat cream, butter

• Nuts and seeds - macadamias, walnuts, sunflower seeds

• Avocado and berries - raspberries, blackberries, and other low glycemic impact berries

• Sweeteners - stevia, erythritol, monk fruit, and other low-carb sweeteners

• Other fats - coconut oil, high-fat salad dressing, saturated fats, etc.

BENEFITS OF A KETOGENIC DIET

When people say that the keto diet changed their life they are not exaggerating. When you decide to switch over to the ketogenic diet, you quickly realize that it is more than just a diet. It's a completely new lifestyle that offers numerous benefits.

Weight Loss

Most people look into a specific diet to lose weight and the keto diet is one of the most effective ways to lose weight in a healthy manner. Because the ketogenic diet is using body fat as an energy source, your body will begin to burn the unwanted fat causing obvious weight loss benefits.

On keto, your insulin (the fat storing hormone) levels drop which allows your fat cells to travel to the liver and get converted into ketones. Your body effectively becomes a fat burning machine.

Control Blood Sugar

Unfortunately, many people suffer from diabetes which is caused by your body's inability to handle insulin. Keto naturally lowers blood sugar levels due to not eating as many carbs so your body can't produce glucose. Keto has been shown to have huge benefits for people that are pre-diabetic or have Type II diabetes. Because the ketogenic diet helps you to maintain more consistent blood sugar levels you find that you have more control of your everyday life while on keto.

Mental Focus

This is one of those benefits that have to be experienced. You can't understand how cloudy carbs make your thinking until you can wean yourself off of them. When on the ketogenic diet you experience increased mental performance.

In fact, many people partake in keto simply for this reason. The reason why you experience an increase in mental performance is that ketones are a great fuel source for your brain. The increase in fatty acids has a huge impact on brain function.

Increase in Energy

You've already learned that keto helps your body turn fat into an energy source. But, did you know that this helps to increase your energy levels? Because your body can only store so much glucose, when it runs out it means your body has run out of fuel (energy) and it needs more. Carbs also cause spikes in blood sugar levels and when those levels drop you experience a crash. Keto helps to provide your body with a more reliable energy source allowing you to feel more energized throughout the day.

Better appetite control

When eating a diet that is heavy in carbs you can often find yourself hungry a lot sooner than you expected after eating a meal. Because fats are more naturally satisfying they end up leaving our bodies in a satiated state for much longer. That means no more random cravings along with feeling like you're going to collapse if you don't get something in you immediately.

Epilepsy

Keto has been used to treat epilepsy since the early 1900s. It's still one of the most widely used treatments for children suffering from uncontrolled epilepsy today. A big benefit of the ketogenic diet for people that suffer from epilepsy is that it allows them to take fewer medications which is always a good thing.

Cholesterol & Blood Pressure

The ketogenic diet has been shown to improve triglyceride levels and cholesterol levels. The benefit? The less toxic buildup in the arteries allowing blood to flow throughout your body as it should. Low carb, high-fat diets show a dramatic increase in HDL (good cholesterol) and a decrease in LDL (bad cholesterol). Studies have shown that low-carb diets show better improvement in blood pressure over other diets.

Because some blood pressure issues are associated with excess weight, the keto diet is an obvious warrior against these issues due to its natural weight loss.

Insulin Resistance

Insulin resistance is the reason why people suffer from Type II diabetes. The ketogenic diet helps people lower their insulin levels to healthy ranges so that they are no longer in the group of people that are on the cusp of acquiring diabetes.

Acne

One of the more common improvements that people on the keto diet experience is better skin.

CHAPTER EIGHT
FOLLOWING THE KETOGENIC DIET

When following the keto diet all these are going to happen

• Lost an average of 3.45 kilograms (7.6 pounds) compared to those in the control group who had no loss in body weight.

• Lost an average of 2.6% body fat while those in the control group did not lose any body fat.

• Lost on average 2.83 kilograms (6.2 pounds) of fat mass (the portion of the body composed strictly of fat) compared to the control group who did not lose any fat mass?

• Maintained lean body mass to the same degree as those in the control group.

• Improved Crossfit performance to the same degree as those in the control group.

• HDL cholesterol (the good one) levels significantly increased.

• LDL cholesterol (the bad one) levels significantly decreased after treatment.

• The level of triglycerides (fat) decreased significantly following 24 weeks of treatment.

• The level of blood glucose significantly decreased.

• An important marker of insulin sensitivity and cardiovascular disease — known as high molecular weight (HMW) adiponectin — significantly increased in the ketogenic diet group but not in the hypocaloric diet group.

SHOULDN'T I BE EATING MORE PROTEIN?

Even on keto, you still want to consume sufficient protein for the benefits: more calories burned at rest (muscle burns fat!) and decreased feelings of hunger because protein is one of the most satiating macronutrients.

That said, the ketogenic diet is not a high-protein diet. Carb and protein intake are both limited so that the body breaks down fat and uses ketones for fuel instead.

You must eat enough protein to maintain muscle mass and organ function, but that's it. If you consistently eat more protein than your body needs, or if both carb and fat intake are low, your body turns protein amino acids into glucose to be used for energy. This is known as gluconeogenesis, which breaks down lean muscle and can raise your blood glucose and insulin levels, thus affecting ketone production. This occurs because your body has an alternate source of glucose so it halts ketone production. A high-protein diet is not ketogenic because you won't be in ketosis. This brings us to the next point: low-carb is also not synonymous with ketogenic.

LOW-CARB IS NOT KETOGENIC

The difference between ketogenic and low-carb diets is that the ketogenic diet aims for ketosis. Other low-carb diets may not have a large enough decrease in carb intake to shift your metabolism into producing and burning ketones for fuel. But, certain types of keto diets do have some leeway with carb and protein intake.

Calculating your macros is essential to achieving your goals.

So what goes into calculating your macros?

Your basal metabolic rate (BMR)

Your BMR is the base number of calories you need to support your body's vital functions (breathing, heart beating, digesting food) without counting the calories needed for daily activities and exercise.

• Your age, gender, height, and weight determine your BMR.

• Weight and height: The bigger you are, the more calories you need so your organs can support you.

• Age: Muscle mass goes down as you age, which can decrease your BMR.

• Gender: Body composition differs between men and women.

We get a close calculation of BMR using the

Harris-Benedict equation:

BMR formula for men = 66 + (6.2 x Weight in pounds) + (12.7 x Height in inches) – (6.76 x Age)

BMR formula for women = 655.1 + (4.35 x Weight in pounds) + (4.7 x Height in inches) – (4.7 x Age)

For example:

A 28-year old woman weighing 130 pounds and standing at 5'2 would calculate her BMR as:

665.1 + 565.1 + 291.4 – 131.6 = 1390 calories needed to support bodily function

A 28-year old man weighing 182 pounds and standing at 6'1 would calculate his BMR as:

66 + 1128.4 + 914.4 − 189.28 = 1919.52 calories needed to support bodily function

• Your total daily energy expenditure (TDEE)

Your TDEE includes all sorts of exercise, whether it's your daily workout or physically demanding days at work or at home. This matters in calculating your calories and macros.

Use these numbers as a guide:

• 1.2: Little to no exercise

• 1.375: Light exercise, 1-3 days per week

- 1.55: Moderate exercise, 3-5 days per week

- 1.725: Hard exercise, 6-7 days per week

- 1.9: Very intense exercise

Which number best matches your activity level? Multiply that number by the BMR number you calculated above. The product is your total daily calorie expenditure or total calorie burn. For example, a woman with a BMR of 1500 who does moderate exercise would have this formula: 1500 x 1.55 to get her total daily calorie expenditure, 2,325. She burns 2,325 calories to support her body and daily activities.

Your body composition: body fat percentage and lean body mass

Your body fat percentage determines your lean body mass — the total weight of your body minus your fat mass — which in turn determines the amount of protein you need to maintain your muscles. This is why most gyms have skinfold calipers, which are surprisingly near-accurate.

Other ways to measure body fat percentage are:

• DEXA scan. This stands for dual-energy x-ray absorptiometry, measures bone mineral density, but can also accurately measure your body fat percentage. It's pricey and can take up to 30 minutes, but it is the gold standard for measuring body fat percentage.

• Body measurements. Apps and online tools provide body fat calculations using your height, weight and the tape measurements of your neck, waist, and hips.

• Photos. Visual estimates provide a more accurate estimate than body measurements. Take a full body photo of yourself and then compare it with the photos of other people. Keep taking photos. It will come in handy later as you track your progress.

Calculating your body fat and lean body mass

Subtract your body fat from your weight and you get your lean body mass.

Convert your body fat percentage into pounds first. For example, your body fat is 25% and you weigh 150 pounds. 150 pounds x .25 = 37.5 pounds of body fat.

Next, subtract that from your weight.

150 pounds – 37.5 pounds of fat = 112.5 pounds of lean body mass.

Save your number. You'll use it later to calculate your protein.

Your weight loss goals

To achieve weight loss, your total calorie intake each day needs to be in a deficit: you consume fewer calories than your total daily expenditure.

A 10%-20% deficit, or even 30% if you can manage, is a good range. Just don't go over a 30%

reduction each day because it can cause long-term issues.

For example, to reduce by 20%, multiply your total calorie expenditure by 0.20. Subtract that amount from your total calorie expenditure. That is your total daily calories, the maximum amount of calories you should consume each day. Eating less than what you burn daily would burn off the weight you want to lose.

Calculating your carbs

On the ketogenic diet, carbohydrates make up 5%-10% of total calories on average. For most people, that's around 20-50 net grams per day.

• Formula: (total calorie intake x % of calories from carbs) / 4

• Multiply your total calories by the percentage of carbs and divide it by 4 to get grams.

• For a total daily calorie intake of 2000 with the ketogenic 5% to 10% carbs, the formula would be:

• 2000 x 0.05 or 0.10 = 100 to 200 calories from carbs

• 200 / 4 = 25g to 50g of carbs each day.

Calculating your protein

On the ketogenic diet, your protein intake should be moderate at about 20% to 25% of your total calories, enough to maintain muscle, but not too much that it affects ketosis. Your protein intake should support your activity level and maintain your lean body mass, which you calculated above.

Calculating your fat

On the ketogenic diet, fat should comprise 70-80% of your total calories. Simply add up your total calories from protein and carbs, then subtract the total from 100 to get your total calories from fat.

100 to 200 calories of carbs + 400 to 500 calories of protein = 500 to 700 calories

2000 total calories − 500 to 700 = 1500 to 1300 calories from fat

Fat has 9 calories per gram so we divide the calories by 9 to get grams. 1500 or 1300 / 9 = 167g or 144g of fat.

The above calculations for your carbs, protein and fat macros give you a range to work in, not guaranteed exact and accurate, but you can adjust. Your body will tell you what it needs and what it likes. Some keto-ers report staying in ketosis in varying amounts of carbs and protein.

Exercising on the keto diet

The well-known formula of eating less and exercising more to lose weight is outdated, untrue and unsustainable. What you eat matters, and the ketogenic diet is one of the tools for weight loss where this is most prominently visible.

Exercise promotes lean muscle building, greater bone strength, and improved stamina and stability. Exercise also uses up your glycogen stores, helping you get into ketosis faster. So look at exercise as a tool to achieve these benefits rather than solely to lose weight.

4 TYPES OF EXERCISE IN KETOSIS

• Aerobic exercises: Cardio. Lasts over three minutes to raise your heart rate. Lower intensity, steady-state cardio is fat burning, making it very friendly for the keto dieter.

• Anaerobic exercises: HIIT or weight training to build muscle. Intense, short bursts of energy to promote strength and speed. Carbohydrates are the primary fuel for anaerobic exercise, so fat alone can't provide enough energy for this type of workout.

• Flexibility exercises: Yoga and stretches, for improving muscle and joint movement, and preventing injuries from the shortening of muscles over time.

• Stability exercises: Core training, Pilates, balance exercises, yoga. Improves alignment, balance, muscle strength and movement control.

Tips

• To use ketones for fat burning:

• Take one scoop of Perfect Keto Base anytime in between meals for constant fat burning.

• To use ketones to get into ketosis (or get back into it after a cheat day):

• Take ½ a scoop of Perfect Keto Base whenever you want to get into ketosis quickly and/or right after a meal that's heavier on carbohydrates than usual.

• To use ketones for energy during the keto transition or fasting:

Before a workout that will be 45 minutes or longer, take a full scoop. Then take another ½ of a scoop for every hour exceeding two hours of continuous work you do. You can take either Perfect Keto Base or Perfect Keto Perform Pre-workout. Note that it's not advised to do heavy workouts while transitioning to keto or during your fast.

Dealing with Weight Loss Plateaus on the Ketogenic Diet

Keto-ers delight in the fast progress they see with the ketogenic diet. There's often a dramatic drop in weight as you lose all those carbs and water weight. The plateau comes next: your weight loss slows way down or even seems to stop as you start losing real fat. You can't seem to break through it no matter how hard you try.

Tips

1 to 2 pounds a week is healthy weight loss. You may be losing gradually, but you're still losing weight. Not losing anything for a week now and then is okay.

Plateaus happen for a reason. Troubleshoot your plateau so you can fix it.

Troubleshooting Your Plateau

Anytime you stop losing weight, see if any of the following could be the reasons and implement the necessary adjustments.

• Are you eating too many carbs?

• Are you missing hidden carbs?

• Are you eating too much protein?

• Are you in ketosis? Do you track your ketone levels often?

• Are you eating too many calories?

• Are you eating quality keto foods?

- Are you eating real, whole foods? Anything packaged could be full of hidden carbs and other artificial fillers.

- Are you eating too many nuts? Not all nuts are made equal, and some could be kicking you out of ketosis and your calorie budget.

- Are you fasting? Intermittent fasting is a great tool for breaking through weight loss plateaus.

- Are you getting closer to your goal weight? The deficit of energy needed for fat loss gets smaller as your weight goes down. You'll keep losing, but it will slow down.

• Are you getting enough sleep?

• Are you managing your stress?

• Are your hormones in good shape? Adrenal or thyroid issues can affect weight loss. Save yourself the frustration and consult your doctor to treat the underlying cause.

During the ketogenic diet, it's crucial that you track. You should be able to answer the above troubleshooting questions with certainty. If not, it means you haven't been tracking properly.

The ketogenic diet induces ketosis, a measurable state of metabolism that can be a great approach to losing weight through fat burning. Because it involves your metabolism, your results will be unique to you, whether or not it's a faster or slower weight loss. The ketogenic diet is a regimen used to treat and manage disease and promote overall health– weight loss is just a bonus. But the healthiness of implementing keto still depends on how you implement it.

CHAPTER NINE
21 DAY KETOGENIC DIET PLAN

TIPS FOR STARTING

Some people don't believe in counting calories on a ketogenic diet, but I am one of the few that does. For most normal people, the amounts of fats and protein will be enough to naturally keep you satiated and naturally keep you in a calorie deficit. Though, the average American is not always normal. There are tons of hormone, endocrine, and deficiency problems that we need to take into account. That said, it doesn't always allow you to lose weight when you are consuming more than your own body is expanding. "Macros" is a shortened version of macronutrients. These are the "big 3" – fats, proteins, and carbs. You can use a calculator to find out how much or how little of each you need in order to attain your goals. You can find the calculator on the navigation bar of the site!

A lot of people take their macros as a "set in stone" type of thing. You shouldn't worry about hitting the mark every single day to the dot. If you're a few calories over some days, a few calories under on others – it's fine. Everything will even itself out in the end.

It's all about a long-term plan that can work for you, and not the other way around. I wanted to put it out there that I made this meal plan specifically with women in mind. I took an average of about 150 women and what their macros were. The end result was 1600 calories – broken down into 136g of fat, 74g of protein, and 20g net carbs a day. This is all built around a sedentary lifestyle, like most of us live. If you need to increase or decrease calories, you will need to do that on your own terms.

To increase calories, it's quite easy – increase the amounts of fat you eat. Olive oil, coconut oil, macadamia nuts, and butter are great ways to increase fats without getting too much of the other stuff in the way. Drizzle it on salads, slather it on vegetables, snack on it, do what you need to do to make it work in your favor!

To decrease calories, you will have to think about what you need. Most likely, you will need less protein as well. So, keep in mind the portions of sizes of meals. Decrease them as you need to, or see fit.

Last, but certainly not least, is sticking to the diet! Ketosis is a process that happens in your body. You can't just have "that one" cheat meal. If you do, it can hamper progress for up to a week before your body is back in ketosis and normally functioning again.

You want to keep your cheats to none. Be prepared, make sure you're eating what you need to be satiated ("full"), and make sure you're satisfied with what you're eating. If you have to force yourself to eat something, it will never work out in the end. This is just a guideline on how you can eat on a ketogenic diet, so you're very welcome to change up what kind of foods you eat!

MEAL PLAN INTRODUCTION

Tried to scale the recipes as best as I could in this meal plan, but not every recipe will be scaled, and some recipes will give leftovers. Make sure you look a few days ahead in the meal plan, as some leftovers are used. Freeze things if you have too many leftovers. You can always re-use this food later on! Some of the food, for example, the Not Your Caveman's Chili, is used in the first week and then again in the last week.

You could use the same batch you cook in the first, which not only saves you energy and time but also saves money. Just freeze it and bring it out to defrost as needed.

I initially intended to keep the net carb count around 20 a day, but it ended up working out even better than that. The 28 day average for the net carbs is 11.2g Net Carbs per day. The total carbs, on average, is 19.6g per day.

Even if you're not counting net carbs, this would be a great way to quickly get yourself into ketosis. Although I wanted to get as close to the macros as I could, I was off by a little bit. The 28 day average across all days comes out to 1597 Calories –

broken down into 136g Fats, 19.6g Carbs, 8.4g Fiber, 11.2g Net Carbs, and 74.9g Protein.

21 DAY KETOGENIC DIET PLAN

WEEK 1 & WHAT TO EXPECT

Our main goal here is to stay pretty simple at first. In my eyes, simplicity is key for someone that is just starting out on a low carb diet. You don't want it to be a difficult transition (kitchen-wise), because it will be hard to just get rid of your cravings.

Leftovers will be another thing we will take into consideration. Not only is it easier on you, but why put yourself through the hassle to cook the same food more than once? Breakfast is something I normally do leftover style, where I don't have to worry about it in the morning and I certainly don't have to stress about it. Grab some food out the fridge, pre-made for me, and head out the door. It doesn't get much easier than that, does it? The first signs of ketosis are known as the "keto flu" were headaches, brain fogginess, fatigue, and the like can really rile your body up.

Make sure that you're drinking plenty of water and

eating plenty of salt. The ketogenic diet is a natural

diuretic and you'll be seeing more than normal.

Take into account that you're peeing out

electrolytes, and you can guess that you'll be

having a thumping headache in no time. Keeping

your salt intake and water intake high enough is

very important, allowing your body to re-hydrate

and re-supply your electrolytes. Doing this will

help with the headaches, if not get rid of them

completely.

If you need to, drink water with a sprinkling of salt in it. Just keep drinking water (I recommend 4 liters a day), and keep eating salt. It will help, trust me. If you're worried about high blood pressure and salt, don't be! Recent studies show that the sodium intake and blood pressure are not as correlated as we so once believed.

Breakfast

For breakfast, you want to do something that's quick, easy, tasty, and of course – gives you leftovers. I suggest starting day 1 on a weekend.

This way, you can make something that will last you for the entire week.

The first week is all about simplicity. Nobody wants to be making breakfast before work, and we're not going to be doing that either.

Lunch

We're also going to keep it simple here. Most of the time, it'll be salad and meat, slathered in high-fat dressings and calling it a day. We don't want to get too rowdy here. You can use leftover meat from previous nights or use easy accessible canned chicken/fish. If you do use canned meats, try to read the labels and get the one that uses the least (or no) additives!

Dinner

Dinner will be a combination of leafy greens (normally broccoli and spinach) with some meat. Again, we'll be going high on the fat and moderate on the protein.

WEEK 2 & WHAT TO EXPECT

Wow, week 1 is over. I hope you're still doing well on the diet and have found it pretty easy breezy to keep on track with everything! This week we're going to be keeping it simple for breakfast again. We're going to introduce ketoproof coffee. It's a mixture of coconut oil, butter, and heavy cream in your coffee. If this repulses you – and I know some of you are saying "WHAT?" – just put some trust in me! This concoction is not as strange as it sounds.

Butter, after all, is made out of cream. So when you blend the oil, butter, and cream together it just adds a decadent richness to your coffee that I am quite sure you'll really like!

Breakfast

For breakfast, we are going to change it up a bit. Here's where we introduce ketoproof coffee. Now, don't get me wrong – I know some of you won't like it. If you're not a fan of coffee, then try it with tea. If you're not a fan of the taste (which is very rare), then try making a mixture of the ingredients by themselves and eating it like that. So, why ketoproof coffee?

Fat Loss. Plain and simple, the consumption of medium-chain triglycerides (MCT) has been shown to lead to greater losses in adipose tissue (fat tissue), in both animals and humans.

Fats! Do I even need to explain this one? Eating fat has been shown to lead to greater amounts of energy, more efficient energy usage, and more effective weight loss. Not to mention, it's the main component of this diet.

More Energy. Studies have shown that the rapid rate of oxidation in MCFAs (Medium Chain Fatty Acids) leads to an increase in energy expenditure. Primarily, MCFAs are converted into ketones (our best friends), are absorbed differently in the body compared to regular oils, and give us more overall energy.

Feel free to add sweetener and spices to this if you're not the biggest fan of the taste. Cinnamon, stevia, vanilla extract. Whatever you'd like to make it great tasting. You can even switch up the taste each and every day so you don't get bored! If this is your first time drinking ketoproof coffee, I suggest taking 1-2 hours or so to drink it down. Normally when people have a large exposure to coconut oil and they're not used to it, it can make them go to the bathroom quite often. Make sure you build a tolerance to coconut oil before drinking it within a 20-minute time frame.

Lunch

We're still keeping simple here. We can incorporate more meat from the previous night of cooking into each lunch we do. Green vegetables and high-fat dressings (or vinaigrettes) are key. Making sure to balance out the fats with the amounts of protein is very important.

Dinner

Dinner, again, will be pretty simplistic. Meats, vegetables, high-fat dressings are the center of our life. Maybe even a slathering of butter on our vegetables since we're getting friskier. Don't over think things in the first 2 weeks; simple is a success.

WEEK 3 & WHAT TO EXPECT

This week we're introducing a slight fast. We're going to get full on fats in the morning and fast all the way until dinner time. Not only are there a myriad of health benefits to this, it's also easier on our eating schedule (and cooking schedule). I suggest eating (rather, drinking) your breakfast at 7 am and then eating dinner at 7 pm. Keeping 12 hours between your 2 meals. This will help put your body into a fasted state. In a fasting state, our bodies can break down extra fat that's stored for the energy it needs. When we're in ketosis, our body already mimics a fasting state, being that we have little to no glucose in our bloodstream, so we use the fats in our bodies as energy.

Intermittent fasting is using the same reasoning – instead of using the fats we are eating to gain energy, we are using our stored fat. That being said, you might think it's great – you can just fast and lose more weight.

You have to take into account that later on, you will need to eat extra fat in order to keep out of a starvation mode state. There are a number of benefits shown that come from intermittent fasting. Some of these include blood lipid levels, longevity, and the much needed mental clarity.

If you find that you can't do a fast, then no big deal. Go back to week 1 and experiment as you see fit. You can eat what you want as long as it fits into your macros.

This is where things start to get more fun – less to worry about, more deliciousness to cook!

Breakfast

We're going full-on fats with breakfast, just like we did last week. This time we'll double the amount of ketoproof coffee (or tea) we drink, meaning we double the amount of coconut oil, butter, and heavy cream. It should come to quite a lot of calories, and should definitely keep us full all the way to dinner. Remember to continue drinking water like a friend to make sure you're staying hydrated.

Lunch

No lunch, oh no! Don't worry – the fats from the morning should keep you feeling energized and full all the way through lunch. Normally people start hitting a wall at first at around 2 pm, so make sure you have plenty of water to drink, drink, and drink.

Dinner

Well, dinner is staying the same. Meats, vegetables, and fats are almost always going to be the dinnertime norm. But don't worry – we'll mix in some bread type things! And guess what, we get to eat dessert this week! Woo! We'll be creating some low carb and great tasting treats that will reward you ever so much for doing the fasting. Sweets, treats, and losing weight – lucky us, right?

Create your own keto diet plan!

You can use my plan as a guideline to help you create something that fits into your life and schedule. Keep in mind that hitting your daily macros is the most important thing when it comes to dieting. Keep in mind that should usually never go above a 15% calorie deficit (to lose weight) or surplus (to gain muscle).

Halloween, Christmas, New Year's Eve, Valentine's day, St. Patrick's day and Easter. These are the holiday seasons where most people would eat, drink and be merry. Most people would gain weight during these seasons. The question is: How to lose weight quick? Everyone else would agree that diet and exercise is the answer. Diet does not necessarily mean not eating anything. It simply means to eat healthily. It is best to read the back of the labels. Check on how much calories, fats, carbs, and sugars each thing that you eat has. Base your food consumption on the serving size. Choose foods that are high in fiber and fewer calories. Choose chicken and fish over pork or beef. Avoid sodas and other high-calorie beverages. Go for water and fruit juices. There are tons of alternatives on how you can enjoy good food without gaining weight. Check out low fat, low-calorie recipes.

Do not overeat. When you are hungry, it will be difficult for you to control how much you can eat. Pack your food in zip lock bags. Do this to control the amount of food that you eat. The amount of calorie you take in should be equal to the amount of exercise that you are ready to do. For starters, do activities that will help you burn 500-700 calories in a day, three times per week. You can eat a more on those 3 days than the 4 days where you don't do exercises. Choose an exercise that you'll enjoy so you'll have fun while losing weight.

It can be basketball, running, rowing, swimming, dancing or kickboxing. All these activities will help you burn calories.

Keep a record of your daily activities, and food intake. Write down all the food that you eat and the calories that you gained. Also, take note of the exercises that you did for the day. Weigh yourself and check your measurements every day. This will help motivate you in reaching your target weight and help you track your progress. Losing weight quickly is easy. All you need to have is some motivation and small changes in your lifestyle. Start working on it now and you'll soon find out that you've already reached your goal.

We shall be discuss on the following

• Chicken Crisps

• Bacon-Wrapped Mini Meatloaf's

• Keto Sandwich Bread

• Waldorf-Stuffed Tomatoes

CHICKEN CHIPS-HOW TO MAKE CHIPS WITH CHICKEN BREAST

chicken chips

Chicken chips is a tasty, tempting and variety appetizer recipe. the outcome of the recipe depends on how you cut the chicken. you need to sharpen the knife before cutting the chicken into pieces. This is the first time I have tried this recipe. felt little nervous while cutting the chicken into very thin layers. but finally, they came out really very nice. I have prepared the chips with very less and common ingredients but you can add seasoning herbs and spices of your choice. like oregano, thyme, parsley, etc while mixing the coating batter.

it tastes good when served with mayonnaise and tomato ketchup.try and enjoys the recipe

Chicken chips-how to make chips with chicken breast

Recipe Type: Appetizer

• Prep time: 30 min

• Cook time: 20 min

• Total time: 50 min

• Serves: 2-3

Ingredients

• Chicken breast – 1

• Corn flour – 1/2 cup

• Water – enough to mix the batter

• Salt – as required

• Red chili powder – 1/2 tsp

• Turmeric powder – a pinch

• Ginger garlic paste – 1/2 tsp

• Oil – for deep-frying

• Sharp slicing knife

Instructions

• Cutting chicken

• Take a sharp meat slicing knife.

• Place your hand on top of the chicken.

• Slice it down from wide end to narrow end.

• Cut each layer as thin as possible.

• Cut the chicken layers into the size of chips.

• Next pound them flat using any heavy object.

Mixing the coating batter

• Take a mixing bowl, add 1/2 cup of corn flour, salt, a pinch of turmeric powder,1/2 tsp of red chili powder,1/2 tsp of ginger garlic paste.

• Pour enough water to make thick pouring consistency batter.

• Put the chicken pieces in the batter.

• Deep-frying.

• Heat oil for deep-frying.

• When the oil is hot, leave chicken pieces into the oil carefully.

• Fry until they turn into nice golden color.

Ingredients

BACON-WRAPPED MINI MEATLOAVES

• 1 small onion (minced, about 1 cup)

• 2 cloves garlic (minced)

• 1 teaspoon fresh thyme leaves (roughly chopped)

• 1 pound ground beef (80/20)

• 1/2 pound ground pork

• 1/2 pound ground veal

• 3 tablespoons Worcestershire sauce

• 1 large egg (beaten)

• 1 cup plain breadcrumbs

• 1/4 cup fresh parsley (roughly chopped)

• 18 slices bacon (1/4 of each piece trimmed off)

• olive oil

• kosher salt and freshly ground black pepper

Directions

Preheat oven to 375ºF. Line a sheet tray with foil and spray it with cooking spray.

Place a sauté pan over medium heat and add a drizzle of olive oil. Add the onion and garlic with a pinch of salt. Cook, stirring occasionally for 3 minutes.

Add the thyme and continue to stir and cook until the vegetables have softened about 2 more minutes. Remove from heat and set aside to cool.

In a large mixing bowl, combine the beef, pork, veal, Worcestershire, egg, breadcrumbs, and parsley. Season with 2 teaspoons of salt and some freshly cracked black pepper.

Add the cooled onion mixture to the bowl and mix to thoroughly combine. Divide the mixture into 6 portions, about ¾ cup each. Form into 6 mini meatloaves. Set aside.

Place 3 pieces of trimmed bacon a clean work surface, overlapping them slightly. Place a mini meatloaf in the center of the bacon slices. Bring the ends of the bacon up on both sides, wrapping the meatloaf. Place bacon-wrapped meatloaf, seam side down, on the prepared sheet tray. Repeat with the remaining meatloaves and bacon. Bake meatloaves for 30-35 minutes, until the bacon, has crisped and the meat is cooked through. (The internal temperature should be 155°F.) Remove from the oven and let rest for 5 minutes before slicing and serving.

KETO SANDWICH BREAD

For those who eat low-carb or keto diets, there is almost always something you can eat at every fast food place or restaurant. Plan ahead. Before entering a restaurant, check out their menu and nutrition information online at home or using your smartphone. It's always good to know the safe options before being tempted by menu items you shouldn't have on a low-carb diet.

In order to make it easier to find a quick keto-friendly option, I've compiled a list of several restaurants and fast food places and those items that I've found to be the lowest carb (and most emotionally satisfying) choices. These are not all perfect options, but when you're stuck with no other choices due to time or location constraints, they'll do in a pinch.

It's a huge help that fast-food places are required to post nutritional content. It gets easier to follow the keto plan every day. The carb count I'm listing is approximate and is NET grams. In general, there is usually some salad option anywhere you are. At Burger joints, just remove the bun, and many places offer lettuce wraps instead. Chicken shouldn't have breading.

As a side note, it helps to have a knife and fork handy in your car or purse. Big, juicy burgers in tiny pieces of lettuce end up on the table - or in your lap. Small, flimsy fast-food plastic ware also makes for difficult eating. Pull out your own sturdy utensils and enjoy!

CONCLUSION

It's difficult if you are just starting out looking for a diet that works for you, to know where the truth lies in this debate; if the scientists can't sort it out then how are you going to? The plain truth is that you'll need to educate yourself, weigh up the arguments, and then follow your own best judgment. My experience has been largely positive but you will, no doubt, have heard of friends having problems on low carbohydrate diets for one reason or another. There is no such thing as a miracle diet and most of them are just variations on a theme but all ketogenic-type diets are based upon a very specific principle and that principle has been demonstrated to induce weight loss in many people. Perhaps you should try to base your opinion on the available evidence and not on anecdotes. It's your body and your health, after all. Whichever low carbohydrate, Atkins-type or ketogenic diet you choose you are going to need some good recipes.

WARNING:

Remember that this is only a guide for informational purposes, we are not responsible for any physical or other damage. In case you wish to practice this type of nutrition, we advise you to contact a doctor.

www.ingramcontent.com/pod-product-compliance
Lightning Source LLC
Chambersburg PA
CBHW061800250726
48657CB00001B/213